Gut health Book for Women

Steps for healthy life, weight loss and hormonal balance.

Dr. Morgan Juliet

Copyright

This book is intended for informational purposes only and is not a substitute for professional medical advice, diagnosis, or treatment. Always seek the advice of your physician or other qualified health provider with any questions you may have regarding a medical condition.

Table of content

Introduction

Comprehensive Guide to Gut Health for Women" is an empowering book tailored specifically for women seeking to optimize their well-being through

improved gut health. In this
enlightening read, you'll embark
on a journey to understand the
intricate connection between your
gut and overall health, exploring
the latest research and practical
strategies. From nurturing a
diverse microbiome to harnessing
the power of probiotics, this book
offers a holistic approach to
wellness, providing invaluable
insights and actionable tips for
women of all ages. Prepare to
discover how a balanced gut can
pave the way to radiant health
and vitality.In a world where
women play multifaceted roles as
caregivers, professionals, and
pillars of strength, their health
often takes center stage.
"Nourish Your Core" is a
transformative guide meticulously
crafted to address the unique
needs and challenges faced by

women on their journey to vibrant health.

Behind every woman's vitality lies a flourishing gut microbiome, a dynamic ecosystem of trillions of microorganisms that play a pivotal role in overall well-being. This book delves deep into the fascinating world of gut health, illuminating the profound influence it wields over everything from digestion and immunity to mood and hormonal balance.

Drawing upon the latest scientific research, Gut health book for women unveils the secrets to cultivating a resilient gut, providing women with a roadmap to nurture their inner garden of health. It unravels the mysteries of prebiotics, probiotics, and the gut-brain connection, offering practical, evidence-based strategies to enhance gut diversity and balance.

But this book is more than just a science lesson; it's a celebration of womanhood. It acknowledges the distinct phases of a woman's life, from adolescence through pregnancy, menopause, and beyond, tailoring advice and recommendations to suit each unique stage.

With the wisdom contained within these pages, women will not only harness the power of their gut for better digestion and energy but also fortify themselves against chronic illnesses and embrace the boundless vitality that comes from within. Gut health Book for women invites you to embark on a transformative journey towards holistic well-being, empowering women to thrive in every aspect of their lives through the nurturing of their core health.

Gut Health

Gut health refers to the overall well-being and proper functioning of the gastrointestinal (GI) tract, which includes the stomach, small intestine, large intestine (colon), and associated organs such as the liver, gallbladder, and pancreas. It's a complex and dynamic system that plays a crucial role in various aspects of our health. Here are key components of gut health:

1. **Digestion**: The primary function of the gut is to break down food into nutrients that can be absorbed and used by the body. This process involves the secretion of digestive enzymes and the mechanical movement of food through the GI tract.

2. **Microbiome**: The gut is home to trillions of microorganisms, including bacteria, viruses, fungi, and other microbes. Collectively, this community of microorganisms is called the gut microbiome. A healthy microbiome is diverse and balanced, with a predominance of beneficial bacteria that aid in digestion, produce essential vitamins, and help protect against harmful pathogens.
3. **Absorption**: The lining of the small intestine contains tiny finger-like projections called villi and microvilli, which increase the surface area for nutrient absorption. Nutrients from food are absorbed into the bloodstream through this lining.

4. **Immune System:** The gut houses a significant portion of the body's immune system. A healthy gut helps maintain a balanced immune response, protecting against infections while avoiding unnecessary inflammation.

5. **Neurological Connection:** The gut and the brain are connected via the vagus nerve and other communication pathways. The gut-brain axis, often known as this link, affects mood, emotions, and cognitive performance.

6. **Hormonal Regulation**: The gut also plays a role in hormone regulation, including the production of hormones related to appetite and metabolism.

7. **Detoxification**: The liver, an organ closely associated with the gut, aids in detoxifying the body by processing and eliminating toxins and waste products.

Gut health can be influenced by various factors, including diet, lifestyle, genetics, and environmental factors. A balanced and diverse diet that includes fiber-rich foods, fermented foods, and a variety of nutrients can support gut health. Additionally, lifestyle factors such as managing stress, getting regular exercise, and avoiding excessive use of antibiotics can contribute to a healthier gut.

Maintaining a healthy gut is essential for overall well-being, as an imbalanced gut can lead to digestive issues, inflammation, and potentially contribute to various health conditions. Research into gut health is ongoing, and it continues to reveal the far-reaching impact of the gut on our overall health and the importance of nurturing this vital system.

Importance of Gut Health in Women

Gut health is of paramount importance in women for several reasons, as it plays a crucial role in various aspects of their overall well-being and addresses specific health needs associated with their gender. Here are some key reasons why gut health is essential for women:

1. **Digestive Health:** Maintaining a healthy gut is fundamental for proper digestion and absorption of nutrients. Women, like men, require essential vitamins, minerals, and nutrients for overall health. A well-functioning gut ensures that these nutrients are efficiently absorbed, supporting optimal bodily functions.
2. **Hormonal Balance:** Gut health can influence hormonal balance in women. The gut microbiome is involved in the metabolism of hormones like estrogen.

An imbalance in gut bacteria can potentially contribute to hormonal disruptions, which may lead to conditions such as polycystic ovary syndrome (PCOS) or irregular menstrual cycles.

3. **Immune System Support:** A significant portion of the immune system resides in the gut-associated lymphoid tissue (GALT). A healthy gut helps support a strong immune response, protecting women from infections and illnesses.

4. **Mood and Emotional Well-Being:** Emerging research suggests a connection between gut health and mental health. The gut-brain axis influences mood and emotions. Women may be more susceptible to mood disorders like anxiety and

depression, making gut health especially important for emotional well-being.

5. **Reproductive Health**: Gut health can indirectly impact reproductive health. A balanced gut microbiome and proper nutrient absorption support overall reproductive function. Additionally, maintaining a healthy weight through good gut health can contribute to fertility.

6. **Hormone Replacement Therapy (HRT):** Women going through menopause and considering hormone replacement therapy need to be mindful of their gut health. HRT can affect the gut microbiome, potentially influencing digestive comfort and overall health.

7. **Bone Health**: Gut health plays a role in calcium absorption, which is

essential for maintaining strong bones. Many women are at risk of osteoporosis, making proper nutrient absorption vital for bone health.

8. **Menstrual Health**: A healthy gut can potentially mitigate the severity of menstrual symptoms like bloating and digestive discomfort.

9. **Pregnancy**: Gut health during pregnancy is important as it can influence both the mother's well-being and the development of the baby's gut microbiome, which can have long-term health implications.

10. **Breastfeeding**: For breastfeeding mothers, maintaining good gut health can affect the composition of breast milk and, in turn, the baby's gut health.

Long-Term Health: Gut health in women can have implications for long-term health, including the risk of conditions like irritable bowel syndrome (IBS), inflammatory bowel disease (IBD), and autoimmune diseases, which disproportionately affect women.

Overall, nurturing gut health through a balanced diet, stress management, and a healthy lifestyle is essential for women to optimize their physical, mental, and emotional well-being. Consulting with healthcare professionals or registered dietitians can provide personalized guidance to address individual gut health needs.

Steps to Gut Health Revival

Reviving gut health is a multi-faceted journey that involves various lifestyle changes and mindful choices. Here are steps to help you on your path to gut health revival:

1. **Diverse Diet:** Incorporate a wide range of fiber-rich fruits, vegetables, whole grains, and legumes into your diet. This diversity supports a thriving microbiome.
2. **Probiotic Foods**: Include fermented foods like yogurt, kefir, kimchi, sauerkraut, and kombucha to introduce beneficial bacteria into your gut.
3. **Prebiotic Foods:** Consume foods high in

prebiotics, such as garlic, onions, leeks, asparagus, and bananas. These nourish your gut bacteria.

4. **Limit Processed Foods**: Minimize highly processed, sugary, and artificial foods, as they can negatively impact gut health.

5. **Reduce Antibiotic Use**: Use antibiotics judiciously, and when prescribed, consider probiotic supplements to mitigate their effects on your gut.

6. **Hydration**: Keep yourself properly hydrated to help gut health overall and digesting.

7. **Stress Management:** Practice stress-reduction techniques like yoga, meditation, or mindfulness, as stress can harm gut health.

8. **Adequate Sleep:** Prioritize quality sleep,

aiming for 7-9 hours per night, as sleep plays a role in gut repair and maintenance.

9. **Regular Exercise**: Engage in regular physical activity to promote gut motility and a balanced microbiome.

10. **Avoid Overuse of Antibiotics**: Use antibiotics judiciously, and if prescribed, consider probiotic supplements to mitigate their effects on your gut.

11. **Limit Alcohol and Tobacco**: Excessive alcohol and tobacco use can harm the gut lining, so it's best to reduce or quit these habits.

12. **Stay Hydrated:** Drink plenty of water to support digestion and overall gut function.

13. **Mindful Eating:** Eat slowly, chew your food

thoroughly, and savor your meals. This aids in proper digestion.

14. **Consult a Healthcare Professional**: If you have persistent gut issues or suspect gut-related problems, consult a healthcare professional or a registered dietitian for personalized guidance and potentially testing.

Remember that gut health is a journey, and results may take time. Be patient and consistent with these steps, as nurturing a healthy gut can have a profound impact on your overall well-being.

The Gut brain connection

The gut-brain connection, often referred to as the gut-brain axis, is a bidirectional communication system between the gastrointestinal tract (the gut) and the central nervous system (the brain). This intricate relationship plays a crucial role in various aspects of health and well-being. Here is a summary of how the gut and brain interact:

1. **Vagus Nerve Communication:** The vagus nerve is a major player in the gut-brain axis. It serves as a communication highway,

allowing signals to pass between the gut and the brain. Information about digestion, nutrient absorption, and gut health is relayed to the brain, influencing mood, emotions, and even cognitive function.

2. **Neurotransmitters**: The gut produces and houses a significant amount of neurotransmitters, such as serotonin and dopamine, which are often associated with mood regulation. Changes in gut bacteria composition can affect the production and function of these neurotransmitters, impacting mood and mental health.

3. **Immune System**: The gut is a significant component of the body's immune system. An imbalance in gut bacteria (dysbiosis) can trigger immune

responses that may affect the brain and contribute to conditions like inflammation, which is associated with various neurological and mental health disorders.

4. **Microbiome Influence**: The gut is home to a diverse community of microorganisms, collectively known as the microbiome. These microbes produce metabolites and molecules that can influence brain function. An imbalanced or unhealthy microbiome has been linked to conditions like anxiety, depression, and even neurodegenerative diseases.

5. **Stress Response**: Stress can affect gut health, and conversely, gut issues can lead to increased stress and anxiety. The gut-brain

axis plays a role in regulating the body's stress response, and chronic stress can disrupt gut function.

6. **Diet and Gut-Brain Connection:** The foods you eat directly impact your gut microbiome, which, in turn, can affect brain function and mental health. A diet rich in fiber and fermented foods can promote a healthy gut and potentially support better mood and cognitive function.

7. **Clinical Implications:** Understanding the gut-brain connection has led to emerging therapies and interventions that target gut health to improve mental health conditions, such as probiotics, prebiotics, and dietary changes.

In summary, the gut-brain connection is a complex and dynamic relationship that influences various aspects of health, including mood, emotions, and cognitive function. It underscores the importance of a balanced diet, stress management, and overall gut health in promoting mental and emotional well-being. Researchers continue to explore this fascinating connection, opening up new avenues for improving both gut and brain health.

A Balanced Gut Health Meal

A balanced diet for gut health should include a variety of foods that support the growth of beneficial gut bacteria, promote digestion, and reduce inflammation. Here's an example of a gut-healthy meal plan for a day:

Breakfast:

- Overnight oats made with rolled oats, almond milk (or any preferred milk), chia seeds, and topped with fresh berries (e.g., blueberries and strawberries).
- A serving of Greek yogurt with honey and a sprinkle of crushed walnuts for added probiotics and prebiotics.
- Green tea or herbal tea for hydration and potential gut health benefits.

Snack:

- Sliced apple or pear with almond or peanut butter for a dose of fiber and healthy fats.

Lunch:

- Grilled chicken or tofu salad with mixed greens, cherry tomatoes, cucumbers, and a variety of colorful vegetables.
- A side of fermented vegetables like sauerkraut or kimchi for probiotics.
- Olive oil and vinegar dressing for healthy fats.

Snack:

- Carrot and cucumber sticks with hummus for a satisfying and fiber-rich snack.

Dinner:

- Baked salmon or a plant-based protein like lentils or chickpeas.
- Quinoa or brown rice as a side for added fiber.
- Steamed broccoli and roasted sweet potatoes for a variety of nutrients and fiber.
- A small serving of fermented dairy or plant-based yogurt for probiotics.

Dessert (optional):

- A small serving of dark chocolate (70% cocoa or higher) for its potential prebiotic effects.
- Herbal tea or decaffeinated tea to aid digestion before bedtime.

Hydration:

- Throughout the day, stay well-hydrated with water or herbal teas. Proper hydration supports digestive health.

Notes:

- This meal plan emphasizes a wide range of colorful fruits and vegetables, whole grains, lean proteins, and sources of healthy fats.
- Greek yogurt, sauerkraut, kimchi, hummus, and dark chocolate provide probiotics and prebiotics.
- Fiber-rich foods like oats, fruits, vegetables, and whole grains support gut motility and beneficial gut bacteria.
- Fermented foods like sauerkraut, kimchi, and yogurt introduce live beneficial bacteria.
- Lean proteins like chicken, tofu, and salmon provide essential amino acids for overall health.
- Omega-3 fatty acids from salmon, walnuts, and olive oil may have anti-inflammatory effects.

Remember that individual dietary preferences and tolerances vary, so you can adapt this example to suit your taste and dietary needs. Additionally, it's essential to maintain portion control and avoid overeating, as moderation is key to a healthy diet and gut health. Consulting a registered dietitian or healthcare professional can provide personalized guidance for your specific gut health goals.

List of food to consume during Gut health

To promote and maintain gut health, it's essential to incorporate a variety of foods into your diet that nourish and support a diverse microbiome. Here's a list of gut-healthy foods to consume:

Fiber-Rich Foods:
- Whole grains (oats, quinoa, brown rice)
- Legumes (beans, lentils, chickpeas)
- Bran cereals
- Berries (blueberries, raspberries)
- Apples and pears (with the skin)

Fermented Foods:

- Yogurt (with live cultures)
- Kefir (fermented milk or plant-based alternatives)
- Kimchi
- Sauerkraut
- Miso
- Tempeh

3. **Probiotic-Rich Foods**:
   - Probiotic supplements (with healthcare professional guidance)
   - Pickles (fermented in brine)
   - Soft cheeses (e.g., Gouda, mozzarella)
   - Buttermilk

4. **Prebiotic Foods**:
   - Garlic
   - Onions
   - Leeks
   - Asparagus
   - Bananas
   - Jerusalem artichokes

- Chicory root

5. **Leafy Greens:**
    - Spinach
    - Kale
    - Swiss chard
    - Collard greens

6. **Nuts and Seeds:**
    - Almonds
    - Chia seeds
    - Flaxseeds
    - Walnuts

7. **Colorful Vegetables**:
    - Carrots
    - Beets
    - Bell peppers
    - Broccoli
    - Sweet potatoes

8. **Herbs and Spices:**
    - Ginger
    - Turmeric
    - Cinnamon
    - Rosemary
    - Thyme

9. **Fruits**:
    - Berries (mentioned earlier)
    - Papaya
    - Pineapple

- Kiwi
10. **Lean Proteins:**
    - Skinless poultry
    - Fish (especially fatty fish like salmon)
    - Tofu
11. **Fats**:
    - Avocado
    - Olive oil (extra virgin)
    - Fatty fish (rich in omega-3 fatty acids)
12. **Tea**:
    - Green tea
    - Herbal teas (peppermint, ginger)

Remember that a diverse diet is key to a healthy gut, as different foods provide various nutrients and promote the growth of different beneficial bacteria. It's also essential to stay hydrated and limit the consumption of highly processed and sugary foods, as they can negatively affect gut health. Tailor your food choices to your dietary preferences and any specific gut health goals you may have.

Fruits to take to enhance Gut health

Incorporating a variety of fruits into your diet can be for gut health, as they provide essential nutrients, fiber, and natural sugars that support a healthy gut microbiome. Here is a list of fruits to consider including in your diet for gut health:

Berries: Blueberries, strawberries, raspberries,

and blackberries are rich in fiber, antioxidants, and polyphenols that can promote gut health. They may also help reduce inflammation.

2. **Apples**: Apples are a good source of soluble fiber, particularly pectin, which can support digestive health by promoting regular bowel movements and feeding beneficial gut bacteria.

3. **Pears**: Pears are another fruit high in soluble fiber, which aids in maintaining gut regularity and supporting the growth of beneficial bacteria.

4. **Bananas**: Bananas contain prebiotic fiber in the form of resistant starch. This type of fiber nourishes beneficial gut bacteria and contributes to a healthy microbiome.

4. **Kiwi**: Kiwi is a fiber-rich fruit that can help with digestion and promote gut regularity. Additionally, it's a good source of antioxidants and vitamin C.
5. **Oranges**: Citrus fruits like oranges are a great source of fibre and vitamin C, which can help with gut health and immunity in general.
6. **Papaya**: Papaya contains the digestive aiding enzyme papain, which aids in digestion. It's also rich in vitamins and antioxidants that benefit overall health.
7. **Mangoes**: Mangoes are not only delicious but also provide dietary fiber and vitamins that contribute to gut health.
8. **Grapes**: Grapes contain natural polyphenols and antioxidants that may help

reduce inflammation in the gut. They are a source of fiber.

10. **Cherries**: Cherries are rich in antioxidants and fiber, which can support digestive health and reduce oxidative stress.

11. **Plums and Prunes:** Plums and prunes are high in dietary fiber and contain sorbitol, which can act as a natural laxative and promote regular bowel movements.

12. **Watermelon**: Watermelon is hydrating and contains fiber, vitamins, and antioxidants that contribute to overall health and digestion.

When incorporating these fruits into your diet for gut health, it's essential to consume a diverse range of fruits to support a variety of beneficial gut bacteria. Aim to eat whole fruits, as the fiber content in the skin and flesh is beneficial for gut health. Additionally, consider pairing fruits with other gut-friendly foods like yogurt or kefir, as these can provide probiotics that further support your gut microbiome.

List of food to prevent during Gut health

When aiming to maintain or improve gut health, it's a good idea to limit or avoid certain foods that can negatively impact your digestive system and the balance of your gut microbiome. Here's a list of foods to consider avoiding or consuming in moderation:

1. **Highly Processed Foods:** Processed foods often contain additives, preservatives, and artificial ingredients that can disrupt gut health. This includes fast food, sugary snacks, and packaged convenience meals.
2. **Excessive Sugar:** High sugar intake can lead to an overgrowth of harmful gut bacteria. Avoid sugary beverages, candy, and excessive consumption of sweets.
3. **Artificial Sweeteners**: A few artificial sweeteners may harm gut flora. Think about reducing the amount of these additives-containing meals and beverages you consume.

4. **Trans Fats:** Trans fats, which are frequently included in processed and fried meals, can cause inflammation and interfere with gut health. Look for trans fats or partially hydrogenated oils on food labels.
5. **Highly Refined Grains**: Foods made with refined grains, such as white bread and white rice, lack the fiber and nutrients that support gut health. Choose whole grains instead.
6. **Fried Foods**: Fried foods can be high in unhealthy fats and are often low in fiber, which can hinder digestion.
7. **Red Meat**: Consuming large amounts of red meat, especially processed meats like sausages and bacon, has been associated with negative

effects on the gut. Choose lean cuts, and think about plant-based protein options.

8. **Alcohol**: Excessive alcohol consumption can harm the gut lining and disrupt the balance of gut bacteria. Moderation is key.

9. **Dairy (for Some Individuals):** Dairy products can be problematic for people with lactose intolerance or dairy sensitivities. In such cases, consider lactose-free alternatives like almond milk or lactose-free yogurt.

10. **Artificial Additives**: Certain food additives and preservatives may have a negative impact on gut health. It's a good practice to read food labels and avoid products with a long list of artificial ingredients.

11. **Spicy and Greasy Foods:** For some individuals, highly spicy or greasy foods can trigger digestive discomfort. It's essential to listen to your body and avoid these if they cause issues.
12. **Large Meals Before Bed:** Eating large, heavy meals right before bedtime can disrupt sleep and digestion. Try to have your last meal at least a few hours before sleep.

Remember that individual tolerance to these foods may vary, and some people may be more sensitive to certain items on this list than others. If you have specific digestive concerns or dietary restrictions, consider consulting a healthcare professional or registered dietitian for personalized guidance on managing your gut health through your diet.

Link between Gut Health and vagus nerve

The vagus nerve, also known as the cranial nerve X, plays a crucial role in the connection between gut health and the central nervous system, particularly the brain. This connection is known as the gut-brain axis, and the vagus nerve is a key component of this complex bidirectional communication system. Here's how the vagus nerve links gut health and the brain:

1. **Bi-Directional Communication:** The vagus nerve serves as a major communication highway between the gut and the brain. It carries information in both directions, allowing signals to pass from the gut to the brain and vice versa.

2. **Gut-to-Brain Communication:** Information from the gut, including signals related to digestion, nutrient absorption, and gut health, is transmitted to the brain via the vagus nerve. This information influences various aspects of brain function, including mood, emotions, and cognitive processes.

3. **Regulation of Digestion:** The vagus nerve plays a significant role in regulating digestion. It controls processes such

as stomach acid production, peristalsis (the rhythmic contraction of the digestive tract), and the release of digestive enzymes.

4. **Immune System Modulation:** The vagus nerve can modulate the immune response in the gut. It helps to regulate the balance between pro-inflammatory and anti-inflammatory responses, which can impact gut health.
5. **Stress Response:** The vagus nerve is involved in the regulation of the body's stress response. It helps to signal the "rest and digest" response, which counteracts the "fight or flight" response triggered by stress.
6. **Mood and Emotions**: The gut-brain axis, facilitated by the vagus nerve, can

influence mood and emotional well-being. The gut produces neurotransmitters like serotonin, which play a role in mood regulation. An imbalanced gut microbiome or gut issues can affect these neurotransmitter levels, potentially contributing to mood disorders like anxiety and depression.

7. **Neurological Disorders:** Research suggests that the gut-brain connection, including vagus nerve function, may be linked to neurological disorders like Parkinson's disease. Changes in gut bacteria can potentially impact the development and progression of these conditions.

8. **Therapeutic Potential:** Understanding the role of the vagus nerve in gut-

brain communication has led to research into therapies that target this nerve, such as vagus nerve stimulation (VNS), to treat conditions like depression and epilepsy.

In summary, the vagus nerve is a critical component of the gut-brain axis, facilitating communication between the gut and the central nervous system. This connection influences various aspects of health, including digestion, immunity, mood, and overall well-being. Nurturing gut health through diet and lifestyle choices can positively impact this intricate relationship and contribute to improved overall health.

Importance of prebiotic and probiotics in Gut health

Prebiotics and probiotics are essential components of maintaining and promoting gut health. They play distinct but complementary roles in supporting the balance and functionality of the gut microbiome. Here's why they are important:

Importance of Probiotics:

Balancing the Microbiome: Probiotics are live beneficial bacteria that, when consumed, can help restore and maintain a balanced gut microbiome. This balance is crucial for overall digestive health.

2. **Digestive Health:** Probiotics assist in the digestion and absorption of nutrients by breaking down food and producing enzymes that aid in this process. They can also help prevent or alleviate common digestive issues like diarrhea, constipation, and irritable bowel syndrome (IBS).

3. **Probiotics can enhance immune function Support for the Immune System:** The gut is home to a sizable percentage of the immune system.by promoting the growth of beneficial gut bacteria, which can help protect against infections and support the body's defense mechanisms.

4. **Reducing Inflammation:**
Some probiotic strains
have anti-inflammatory
properties, which can be
beneficial in managing
inflammation-related
conditions, such as
inflammatory bowel
disease (IBD) and certain
autoimmune disorders.

5. **Mood and Mental Health:**
Recent studies point to a
link between good gut
health and mental
wellness. Probiotics may
play a role in improving
mood and reducing
symptoms of anxiety and
depression.

Importance of Prebiotics:

1. **Feeding Beneficial
Bacteria:** Prebiotics are

non-digestible fibers that serve as a food source for beneficial gut bacteria. They promote the growth and activity of these bacteria, helping them thrive in the gut.

2. **Enhancing Microbiome Diversity**: A diverse gut microbiome is associated with better health outcomes. Prebiotics encourage the growth of various bacterial species, contributing to a more diverse and robust microbiome.

3. **Improved Digestion:** Prebiotic fibers can help regulate bowel movements and prevent constipation by adding bulk to the stool and promoting regularity.

4. **Nutrient Absorption**: By improving the health and diversity of the gut microbiome, prebiotics can enhance the absorption of

essential nutrients, such as calcium, magnesium, and certain vitamins.

5. **Supporting Overall Health:** A healthy gut microbiome has far-reaching effects on overall health. It can help maintain a healthy weight, reduce the risk of chronic diseases, and support optimal immune function.

In summary, probiotics and prebiotics work together to promote gut health. Probiotics introduce beneficial bacteria into the gut, while prebiotics provide the nourishment these bacteria need to thrive. A balanced combination of both can contribute to improved digestion, better immune function, reduced inflammation, and overall well-being. It's important to note that individual responses to probiotics and prebiotics can vary, so it's advisable to consult with a healthcare professional or registered dietitian for personalized guidance.

Type of exercises you can do

A variety of exercises can contribute to better gut. It's important to engage in regular physical activity that you enjoy and that fits your fitness level and preferences. Here are some types of exercise that can support gut health:

Aerobic Exercise:
Brisk Walking: Walking is a low-impact aerobic exercise that's accessible to almost everyone. Aim for at least 30

minutes of brisk
walking most days
of the week.
Running: Running
or jogging can
provide a more
intense aerobic
workout, which can
help stimulate gut
motility.
2. **Strength Training:**
Weightlifting:
Resistance training
with weights or
resistance bands
can help build
muscle and support
overall metabolism,
which indirectly
influences gut
health.
Bodyweight
Exercises:
Exercises like push-
ups, squats, and
planks are effective
for strength training
and can be done

without any
equipment.

3. **Yoga**:

   - Yoga: Yoga
     combines physical
     postures, breathing
     exercises, and
     mindfulness, which
     can help reduce
     stress and promote
     relaxation,
     benefiting gut
     health.

4. **Pilates**:

   - Pilates: Pilates
     focuses on core
     strength, flexibility,
     and balance, which
     can contribute to
     improved posture
     and abdominal
     muscle tone,
     potentially
     benefiting digestion.

5. **High-Intensity Interval Training (HIIT):**

   - HIIT exercises
     contain short bursts

of intense exercise followed by quick recovery periods.These workouts can provide a time-efficient way to improve cardiovascular fitness and metabolism.

6. **Cycling**:

Cycling: Whether outdoors or on a stationary bike, cycling is an excellent aerobic exercise that can be gentle on the joints.

7. **Dance**:

Dancing: Dancing is a fun and engaging way to get your heart rate up while also improving coordination and balance.

8. **Swimming**:

- . Swimming is a full-body exercise that is gentle on the joints. It can improve cardiovascular fitness and promote relaxation.

9. **Tai Chi**:
   - Tai Chi: This mind-body practice involves slow, flowing movements and deep breathing.It can reduce stress and improve balance.

10. **Hiking**:
    - Hiking: If you enjoy the outdoors, hiking is an excellent way to combine physical activity with nature, reducing stress and promoting overall well-being.

Remember to start slowly, especially if you're new to exercise or haven't been active for a while. Gradually increase the intensity and duration of your workouts to avoid overexertion its also essential to stay hydrated before, during, and after exercise, as proper hydration is crucial for digestion and overall health.

The key is to find activities that you enjoy and can sustain over time. Consistency in your exercise routine is more important than the specific type of exercise you choose when it comes to promoting gut health.

Importance of exercise in Gut health

Exercise can have a positive impact on gut health, although the direct mechanisms are still an active area of research. Engaging in regular physical activity can contribute to a balanced and thriving gut microbiome and promote overall digestive wellness. Here's how exercise can benefit gut health:

Enhanced Gut Motility: Physical activity, especially aerobic exercise, can stimulate gut motility, helping to move food and waste through the digestive tract more efficiently. This can aid in preventing constipation and promoting regular bowel movements.

2. **Reduced Inflammation**: Exercise has been shown to reduce chronic low-grade inflammation, which can be associated with certain gut conditions like inflammatory bowel disease (IBD). By reducing inflammation, exercise may help manage these conditions.

3. **Diverse Gut Microbiome:** Regular exercise has been linked to a more diverse gut microbiome. A diverse microbiome is often associated with better gut health and a reduced risk of gastrointestinal issues.

4. **Improved Insulin Sensitivity**: Physical activity can enhance insulin sensitivity, which can indirectly benefit gut

health. Better blood sugar regulation is associated with a healthier gut environment.

5. **Stress reduction:** Exercise is known to help people feel less stressed and anxious to prevent exhaustion, high stress levels can negatively affect gut health, so managing stress through exercise can be beneficial.

6. **Weight Management:** Maintaining a healthy weight through regular exercise can positively influence gut health. Obesity is associated with alterations in gut microbiota, and exercise can help in weight management.

7. **Release of Short-Chain Fatty Acids (SCFAs):** Exercise may increase the production of SCFAs in the gut, which are beneficial

compounds associated
with improved gut health
and reduced inflammation.

To incorporate exercise into your
routine for better gut health:

1. **Aim for Regularity:**
   Consistency matters. Try
   to establish a routine of
   regular physical activity,
   whether it's daily walks,
   weekly gym sessions, or
   home workouts.
2. **Variety of Activities:**
   Incorporate a mix of
   aerobic exercises (like
   walking, running, or
   cycling) and strength
   training exercises (such as
   weightlifting or bodyweight
   exercises) to support
   overall health.
3. **Stay Hydrated:** Proper
   hydration is crucial for
   digestion. Drink water

before, during, and after
exercise to maintain good
hydration levels.

4. **Listen to Your Body**: Pay
close attention to how
exercise affects your body.
If you experience digestive
discomfort during or after
exercising, consider
adjusting the timing or
intensity of your workouts.

5. **Combine with a
Balanced Diet**: Exercise
complements a healthy
diet for optimal gut health.
Consider combining your
exercise routine with a diet
rich in fiber, fruits,
vegetables, and whole
grains.

Remember that individual
responses to exercise can vary,
so it's essential to find an
exercise regimen that works for
you and consult with a healthcare
professional or fitness expert if

you have specific concerns or
medical conditions

Importance of a calm mind in improving your Gut health

Calming the mind is important for improving gut health because of the intricate connection between the brain and the gut, known as the gut-brain axis. This connection allows for bidirectional communication between these two systems, and a calm mind can positively influence gut health in several ways:

Stress Reduction: Chronic stress can have a significant negative impact on gut health. When you're stressed, your body's fight-or-flight response is activated, which can lead to changes in gut motility, increased inflammation, and alterations in gut bacteria. Calming the mind through relaxation techniques like meditation, deep breathing, and mindfulness can help reduce stress and mitigate its harmful effects on the gut.

2. **Balanced Digestion**: A calm and relaxed state of mind promotes optimal digestion. Stress and anxiety can disrupt the digestive process, leading to issues like indigestion, bloating, and altered bowel movements. When you're relaxed, your body can focus on digesting food more effectively, supporting gut health.

3. **Influence on Gut Permeability:** Chronic stress and anxiety can contribute to increased gut permeability, often referred to as "leaky gut." This condition allows harmful substances to pass through the intestinal lining into the bloodstream, potentially triggering inflammation and immune responses. Calming the mind may help maintain the integrity of the gut barrier and reduce the risk of leaky gut.

4. **Microbiome Balance:** Stress can affect the composition of the gut microbiome, potentially leading to an imbalance between beneficial and harmful bacteria. A balanced, diverse microbiome is associated with better gut health. Calming practices may

help support a healthier gut microbiome.

5. **Improved Eating Habits**: A calm mind can promote mindful eating, which involves paying attention to your food, savoring each bite, and eating without distractions. This can lead to healthier food choices and better digestion, as opposed to stress-induced emotional eating or hurried, unhealthy eating habits.

6. **Positive Mood and Well-Being:** Calming the mind through relaxation techniques can improve mood and reduce symptoms of anxiety and depression. A positive emotional state is associated with better gut health and overall well-being.

7. **Pain Management:** In conditions like irritable

bowel syndrome (IBS),
stress and anxiety can
exacerbate symptoms.
Calming the mind may
help manage pain and
discomfort associated with
gut disorders.

Incorporating stress-reduction
techniques into your daily routine,
such as meditation, mindfulness,
yoga, or deep breathing
exercises, can be beneficial for
both mental and gut health.
Reducing chronic stress and
promoting relaxation not only
supports a healthy gut but also
contributes to overall physical
and emotional well-being.

Conclusion

In conclusion, gut health is of paramount importance for women's overall well-being and vitality. It's a dynamic and interconnected system that impacts various facets of health, from digestion to immune function and even mood regulation. Nurturing your gut health can be a transformative journey, particularly tailored to the unique needs and challenges faced by women at different stages of life.

By embracing a diverse and balanced diet rich in fiber, prebiotics, and probiotics, women can support the flourishing of beneficial gut bacteria and ensure optimal digestion. Mindful choices in nutrition, coupled with stress management techniques like yoga and meditation, can help mitigate the negative impact of chronic stress on gut health.

The gut-brain connection underscores the significance of a calm mind in promoting gut health. Practices that reduce stress and anxiety not only support emotional well-being but also contribute to a harmonious gut environment.

Furthermore, regular physical activity complements dietary efforts, aiding in gut motility and overall metabolic health. Whether through brisk walks, strength training, or relaxation exercises, incorporating exercise into your routine can positively influence gut health.

In essence, taking proactive steps to enhance gut health can empower women to thrive in every aspect of life. It's an investment in long-term well-being, from supporting digestive comfort and immune resilience to fostering a positive mood and overall vitality. Consultation with healthcare professionals or registered dietitians can provide personalized guidance on optimizing gut health, ensuring that women can achieve and maintain vibrant health at every stage of life.

www.ingramcontent.com/pod-product-compliance
Lightning Source LLC
Chambersburg PA
CBHW050846260726
48660CB00006B/2477